PRAISE FOR *INNOVATION WEIGHT LOSS PROGRAM*

Believe in yourself and the program and you will see the results.

"I was so skeptical. How could I possibly lose weight with a cheat day? Won't I gain it all back after I cheat? But Josephine said, 'Follow the program 100% and trust in it.' That's exactly what I did, and she was so right. It changed my life. Not only did I lose the weight but I kept it off. The program helped me lose the weight and I maintain with it too. The program really works. So many of my family and friends are on it and have all done amazingly. You need to trust in it and learn from it. I lost 20 pounds and have never felt better."

—Danya T.

D0937631

Don't let your age or your repeat failures stop you from trying Cheat Day Rules!

"When Josephine told me that my weight was aging me, I knew she was right. I had fallen back on the excuses of 'I'm 65, what does it matter?' and 'I can't look like I did when I was 30.' After learning to live the Innovation program, not only am I thinner than I was when I was 30, but I look and feel better because I'm eating healthy and clean. I lost 44 pounds and feel younger than I have in years. I can't believe I was willing to settle because of my age. Thank goodness I found this program and I found Josephine."

—Kathy A.

You can drop 10 pounds in a week if you really stick to the program.

"I couldn't believe it when Josephine told me that if you follow exactly what is on the menu and don't incorporate anything else you would lose 10 pounds in a week. It was shocking because there are plenty of food choices on the menu. It's not like I was starving. She told me you won't lose it every week, but the majority of people lose 7 to 10 pounds in the first week; and sure enough, I did. Since it was all I needed to lose, I continued on the program and lost another 5 pounds and now I maintain with the program. It really is a way of life. I would never go back to my old habits, and with the cheat day, I don't have to."

—Steve K.

Don't just do the program. It's not a quick fix or fad diet. You need to live the program. It's truly something you can do forever.

"After being on every diet out there, I found this program and realized this is what I needed. It's not a quick fix, it's a way of life; and the cheat day helps me lose the weight and stay on program. I love eating clean on my program days and I love my cheat day. I lost 40 pounds and have kept it off for five years!"

—Susan T.

When you understand how easy this program is, there are no excuses that will work.

"You follow your menu and you lose the weight. It's that simple. I almost let myself use my kids, my job, and lack of time to keep me in a very unhappy place. While I loved everything in my life, my weight was making me miserable every morning. I couldn't even get dressed for work. I refused to keep buying clothes but the ones I had were tight. I looked like a stuffed sausage. When I heard about the Innovation Program, I thought it was too good to be true. How could I possibly lose weight without even meeting Josephine? Sure enough, she gave me all the tools I needed, and not only have I lost the weight, but I feel like I know her, and I love her. She has changed my life. I lost 33 pounds. I still had to buy clothes because all my small clothes didn't fit me. But that was a problem I was happy to have."

—Rita G.

If you can jump out of bed and put your skinny jeans on and they are loose—everything else in the world is okay!

"I loved it when I read one of Josephine's blogs and she talked about if you can jump out of bed and put your skinny jeans on and they are loose—everything else in the world is okay! I thought it's so true. She wrote that everything starts with how you feel, and how you feel starts with how you treat your body. When you are happy and feel good about yourself, that's how you make everyone feel around you. This changed my thinking. I wanted to be the happy person, the person who people want to be around, not the one who was always miserable, complaining about her weight. After reading Josephine's blogs, I started her program and it changed my life. I lost all the weight I wanted and, more importantly, I could see how my attitude changed, because I was happy and it really did change my family. Because I was happy, they were happy. And just like Josephine said, that was all in my control. If I wanted to be happy, I had to work for it. I did it and I love my life, and my family and friends love the new me.

—Gina R.

Enjoy the journey. Sometimes we get so rushed with getting the weight off, we don't enjoy the journey getting to our goal.

"My first week I lost 6 pounds and then I lost anywhere from 1 to 3 pounds per week. After losing the first 10 pounds, all I could think of is I had 40 more to go. It was so hard because you just want it all off at once. But Josephine told me to enjoy the journey. She said you are eating (not starving), you are cheating one day every week, and you are losing every week. Of course, we want it off yesterday; but instead of looking only at the long-term goal, we should have short-term goals too. When I get to 15 pounds, I'm going to feel great, and after I reach 20 I will feel amazing. While 40 is my ultimate goal, I can't forget to enjoy the weight loss along the way. I not only reached my 40-pound weight-loss goal, I loved every minute of it."

—Sara R.

Short-term goals lead to long-term goals.

"For me it was a difficult task to see the number that was on the scale. I couldn't figure out how I got there. Somewhere along the path of kids, family, and work, my weight shot up over 200 pounds. It was so scary to see. While most people didn't even realize it bothered me, Josephine knew right from the beginning. She told me not to focus on where the number was, but look at where it was going. At 209 pounds, our first goal was to get it out of the 200s. We did and it was so much faster than I could ever have hoped. Then we focused on the 190s and getting to the 180s. Just looking for the next second digit made all the difference to me. Before I knew it, I was down 20, then 30. Now reaching my goal of 128 pounds, I am at a number I could never imagine possible. The funny thing is that I didn't even realize the total number because most of the time I was so focused on just seeing the next digit. It became a challenge and one that I loved. I have maintained this weight for two years and every day I get dressed, I just can't believe that I did it. Thank you, Josephine. I owe my life and happiness to you."

—Tina S.

"I'm a private guy. Or at least I used to be. I didn't even want anyone to know I was doing the program. Looking back now, I realize it was because I was afraid of failing and I didn't want the pressure. I was also what I considered private because I was embarrassed about the way I looked. When I saw the pounds come off, I couldn't believe what dropped with it. My cholesterol, my blood pressure, and my sugars all went to normal levels. I could not believe how easy the program is and quickly realized this was my new way of life. I never wanted to be the over-weight guy that was so unhealthy inside and out. I love the way I eat and look and feel—not only do I recommend the program to everyone, so does my Doctor!"

—Josh R.

CHEAT DAY
RULES!

CHEAT DAY RULES!

How to Win at the Weight-Loss
Game by Eating Whatever You
Want One Day a Week

JOSEPHINE FITZPATRICK

Founder of Innovation Weight Loss Program

RADIUS BOOK GROUP
NEW YORK

Distributed by Radius Book Group
A Division of Diversion Publishing Corp.
443 Park Avenue South, Suite 1008
New York, NY 10016

www.RadiusBookGroup.com

Cheat Day Rules! is intended as a reference book only, not as a medical manual. The information given here is designed to help you make informed decisions about your health. It is not intended as a substitute for any treatment that may have been prescribed by your doctor or other health care professional. If you suspect that you have a medical problem, we urge you to seek competent medical help.

For more information, email info@diversionbooks.com.

First edition: January 2018

Paperback ISBN: 978-1-63576-372-0
eBook ISBN: 978-1-63576-373-7

To my amazing husband who is my rock and bulldog

My beautiful children you are my breath and sunshine

My dedicated staff for always giving me your all

To all my fabulous clients for your trust and loyalty

I love you all . . .

CONTENTS

PREFACE

Quick fixes and fad diets? Not a chance. As a weight-loss and nutrition specialist to A-list celebrities, I am all about healthy weight loss, and I prove it by boasting an incredible 99 percent success rate. My program is based on the unique idea that sustainable weight loss never comes from eliminating the foods you love. Instead, I base the weight-loss plan on my personal nutrition philosophy: six days of clean eating, one day of cheating. By creating a balance, my plan allows clients to eat what they love and still lose weight without the risk of dangerous rebounds and splurges. For more than 15 years, I have dedicated myself to helping others achieve their ideal bodies, giving them the tools and guidance they need to lead their healthiest lives.

I began my personal wellness journey at the age of 16 when my father was diagnosed with type 2 diabetes. The severity of the disease eventually led to the amputation of several of his limbs, a tragic event that left me more determined than ever to help people live and eat in a healthier way. At a young age, I was amazed to learn that even foods that are generally considered to be healthy, such as fruits, could have such a negative impact on the body. From some amazing doctors who took the time to teach me at such a young age, I learned that the body processes the natural sugars found in food in the same manner as processed sugars. From that moment on, I dedicated myself to studying nutrition and adopted my new personal motto: "Just because a food is considered healthy doesn't mean it's beneficial for weight loss."

I began my career working as a private nutrition and weight-loss consultant, offering my clients support 24/7 and helping them to find a healthier, cleaner way of life that they could maintain long term. As popularity grew, I launched my unique weight-loss program, offering clients my signature personalized program and support in both my Woodbury, Long Island, and New York City locations. The program was a huge hit, earning thousands of clients in person and online, including high-profile clients and A-list celebrities. You can find us online at any of these URLs: innovationweightloss.com, innovationweightlossandfitness.com, or cheatdayrules .com. The program now boasts an incredible 99 percent success rate, proving that my dedication to balance and maintenance earns real, transformative results.

Following the incredible success of my program, I launched Innovation Foods, a line of delicious, natural foods made with no GMOs, preservatives, or chemicals. Our products make it easier for people to make healthier eating choices, even when they don't have the time to cook, by offering snacks and meals that are freshly prepared each day. You can shop locally at our Woodbury location—or if you need overnight shipping, you can order online at innovationweightloss.com.

I meet with hundreds of clients a month. I hear the stories of how my clients became overweight, the accounts of how impossible it was for them to lose weight, the desire that they have to lose weight, and the need to be the person they once were or always wanted to be. The stories are real. They are of everyday people like you and me. Some are high-profile actors and actresses; some are mothers, fathers, sisters, brothers; they are young and old, and somewhere in-between.

Today in the U.S., there are more overweight and obese children and adults than ever before. Obesity became an epidemic, in part, because of the quick fixes and short-term plans trying to combat years of supersizing foods, including fat-free and no-carb diets, and the now very popular gluten-free diets. The result is millions of yo-yo dieters—people losing weight, then gaining back more than what they originally lost. If you are one of the millions who have gotten caught up with quick fixes and fad diets, then it's time for you to learn how to eat clean to lose weight with real, everyday foods.

INTRODUCTION

W ith the *Innovation Weight Loss Program*, you don't have to say no to the foods you love. You only have to wait until your once-a-week Cheat Day. With the *Innovation Weight Loss Program*, you learn to fuel your body for six days a week for weight loss and health, then take one day to indulge. It would be unrealistic to think that you are never going to eat all the foods you love ever again. On the *Innovation Weight Loss Program*, you don't have to be unrealistic. You just have to be patient. Instead of never, you only have to wait until your once-a-week Cheat Day arrives. My Cheat Day Program has a 99 percent success rate because it teaches you how to successfully use a Cheat Day to lose weight.

To be successful with the *Innovation Weight Loss Program*, start by reading the entire book. I find that sometimes people are so excited to begin that they jump ahead because they just want to start and get the weight off. If you did that, go back and read from the beginning. To do the program successfully, it's important to learn and understand the *Cheat Day Rules!* Once you have read the entire book, then you can begin.

If you have been stuck in fad diets and quick fixes, you have probably experienced a constant cycle of losing and gaining the same pounds repeatedly. The emotional battle involved in this endless cycle of disappointment causes people to fail with their weight-loss quests. Your body needs foods from all food groups—carbohydrates (carbs), protein, and even fats. The only way to create long-term weight loss for a lifetime and a healthy way of eating is to create a balance that works for you.

With my *Innovation Weight Loss Program*, you will never have to count calories again. You'll fuel your body six days a week for weight loss, and then indulge in your favorite foods on your Cheat Day. It's so much easier to stick with a healthy diet when you know that your Cheat Day is just 48 to 72 hours away. Once you learn this new way of eating and living, you'll lose weight and you'll no longer have to say no to foods you love. Millions of people play the weight-loss game every year. Their goal is to get the weight off and keep it off, but the biggest obstacle comes from struggling to stay in the game while fighting—and often giving into—temptation.

If you have tried unsuccessfully and failed to lose weight and keep it off, then *Cheat Day Rules!* is for you. Once you discover this new way of eating, you will never have a weight problem again.

RULE 1

STAY ON PROGRAM FOR SIX DAYS EVERY WEEK

Myth: Going on a diet means I will never be able to eat the foods I love again.

Truth: With Cheat Day Rules, you can eat any or all of your favorite foods one day a week.

E very Monday morning, millions of people start a new weight-loss plan with the best intentions. What diet will it be this time? The low-carb one? A Paleo Diet plan? A raw foods diet? Some other fad-of-the-month diet you read about in a magazine or on a blog? Sound familiar? According to Livestrong.com, the Boston Medical Center indicates that approximately 45 million Americans diet each year and spend $33 billion on weight-loss products in pursuit of trimmer, fitter bodies. For the first few days on any diet, you feel great and are determined to stick with it, but by Thursday or Friday, you're hungry, sleepy, lethargic, and grouchy. After a week of following the diet, you may gain, rather than lose, two to three pounds. You throw in the towel and give up. Why do you keep doing this to yourself? Because you don't know any other way to lose weight.

The first *Innovation Weight Loss Program* rule is that six days a week you fuel your body with healthy, satisfying foods to lose weight, and then on the seventh day, you can indulge and eat whatever you want. That's right, you can eat anything you want one day a week. Knowing that your Cheat Day is just 48 or 72 hours away makes it easier to stick with the *Innovation Weight Loss Program*.

The *Innovation Weight Loss Program* allows you to satisfy your cravings without beating yourself up because you went off your diet. Let's face it: We spend a lot of time deciding what to eat, especially when trying to lose weight. Your Cheat Day is the one day of each week when you don't have to think about what you are eating.

Rule 1 means, however, that you must be focused and vigilant about what you eat on the other six days of the week.

The only way the *Innovation Weight Loss Program* works is if you eat the specific foods as outlined for six days. The program is six days on program, followed by one Cheat Day. I repeat this frequently throughout the book because I want you to know how important it is. While the thought of a Cheat Day is exciting and liberating, you need to stay focused on your weight-loss days—the other six days of the week. If you eat on program, you will lose weight every week.

WHAT DOES EATING "ON PROGRAM" MEAN?

Eating "on program" means eating only the foods listed on the daily menu to help you lose weight. When you follow the menu exactly, you will lose weight and reach your goals of looking and feeling better than ever before. The menu is designed so that you can dine out, order in, or cook at home.

Strategies to Get You through Six Days of Eating on Program

- **Eat when you want.** It doesn't matter if you eat breakfast at noon or enjoy your lunch menu at dinner. You can eat all three snacks at 3 p.m. or 9 p.m., or space them out during the day. What *does* matter is the amount and kind of foods you consume in one 24-hour period. If you force yourself to eat breakfast when you are not hungry, it will not make you less hungry later in the day. If you start your day with coffee, but don't get hungry until noon, then that is when you should eat. If you are not hungry until noon, then do not eat until then. But if you wake up hungry and force yourself not to eat until 12, then you are setting yourself up to overindulge and binge because by the time you eat, you will be starving. If you're not hungry early in the day, then don't force yourself to eat. If you are hungry, then eat your meal. Keep it simple and listen to your body.

- **Get uninterrupted sleep.** Don't get up in the middle of the night and have a few tablespoons of ice cream. Your body and your brain require at least seven hours of sleep every night to recharge and rest. You need sleep, not food, during the night.

- **Learn to recognize when you are bored.** One of my clients told me, "I am starving at night. I want to eat everything." I insisted that he wasn't starving because he ate the three meals and three snacks on the plan throughout the day. He finally conceded that he was bored, rather than hungry. Most people have no trouble following the program during the day because they're so busy, but when they get home, they find themselves looking for treats and snacks. If this sounds familiar, then save your three daily snacks and eat them during the evening.

- **Learn to recognize hunger.** Many of us have access to so much food and so much temptation that we don't know what real hunger feels like. Just the thought of being hungry for some people is beyond what they think they can handle. As soon as they have that little uncomfortable feeling, they immediately feel the need to feed it. Ask yourself, am I really hungry—or am I thirsty, bored, tired, or upset?

• **Avoid preventive eating.** Let's say you're going to the movies or a concert. You're not in the least bit hungry, but your brain tells you that you will be hungry in a couple of hours. To prevent yourself from becoming ravenous, you eat a meal or a snack that you don't really want. The next time this happens, ask yourself if you are truly hungry. My guess is that you are not. Don't eat when you are not hungry. Bring a snack or plan a meal for later. Remember, it's okay to allow yourself to be a little hungry.

Everything Matters: Vegetables Are Not Free Foods

If you eat vegetables, they matter. When clients first come to me, many often think there are *free foods*, like fruits and vegetables, they can consume in endless quantities and lose weight. When I explain that there are no free foods, they start to panic: "What am I going to eat? Can I do this?" If you are thinking the same thing, I want you to know that you can do this! You don't need to, or shouldn't want to, have something in your mouth all the time. Nothing is unlimited, intentionally, and everything you eat matters for a reason.

Eating on program and following your menu 100 percent are not enough when it comes to weight loss. An important tenet you must remember is this: Everything matters and everything counts. If you eat something, whether it's a bagel or broccoli, it matters. There are no free foods on the *Innovation Weight Loss Program*.

When you can't have unlimited vegetables, you are training your brain that you don't need to eat every five minutes. You will stop eating all day long. What happens when all those free vegetables are no longer satisfying? By now you are so used to nibbling all day that you need something to replace those vegetables. When you can eat free foods, you don't learn how to eat and be satisfied with your meals and snacks. You don't learn how to live not putting something in your mouth whether you are hungry or not. Without free foods, you'll learn how to get through the day with your meals and snacks, and realize how quickly you will lose the desire to eat all day long.

Start by recognizing that every bite matters, even half a chicken nugget and a spoonful of mashed potatoes you swiped from your child's plate. Steamed broccoli and grilled fish are a good weight-loss meal. But when you smother the broccoli with Parmesan cheese, or bathe the fish in butter sauce, it's no longer a weight-loss meal. Once you start to understand that every bite, sip, crumb, and piece of anything you eat really does matter, you will see the difference in what you thought you were consuming compared to what you are actually eating. When you think "I hardly ate anything all day," is that true? Or did you have a handful of M&M's and an iced latte that you forgot to count? When it comes to weight loss, everything that passes your lips shows up on the scale.

Everything matters; it is important to understand and control this concept. This is a life-changing concept when it comes to weight loss. It is about realizing that you need to be aware of what you are doing and what is important to you. You will be encouraged to think about whether or not you really *need* a snack at the moment you *want* it, because once you eat it, then it's one less snack you have for the day. When you have free food, like unlimited vegetables, then you don't have to think about it. If you get hungry, you just keep eating vegetables for the remainder of the night. That's not learning how to eat for weight loss; that is continuing a cycle of mindless eating. That's why we have such an obesity epidemic in the U.S. today. Not because vegetables cause obesity, but the need to feed all day surely does.

Learning that everything matters helps you make mindful decisions, such as, "Is it worth that bite? Do I really need to taste that?" A big part of the *Innovation Weight Loss Program* is learning to live with what your body needs, rather than feeding the habit of eating just to eat. Allowing free food gives you the opportunity and excuse to eat mindlessly, whether you are hungry or not. Free foods take away your control—the control you need to learn that you should only be eating when you are hungry, not because you are bored, tired, or stressed.

MENTAL VS. PHYSICAL HUNGER

. . . .

Myth: Ninety percent of the time, we are eating because we are hungry.

Truth: Ninety percent of the time, when we are eating, we are *not* hungry.

. . . .

When it comes to your six clean-eating days, you need to constantly ask yourself, am I hungry? Many times when we reach for a snack, it's because we hear a growl in our tummy or the clock says it's midafternoon. Is the snack what your body wants or is it just something to do at the time? The next time you have a snack attack, ask yourself these questions before you reach for something you don't need and may not even want:

- **Am I thirsty?** Nine out of ten times we are more thirsty than hungry. When we do not properly hydrate, our skin becomes dry and our lips chapped. But when we are thirsty, we tend to reach for food rather than water. Most of the time we do this because we don't even realize that we are thirsty and not properly hydrated. So the next time you think it's time for a snack, drink 8 ounces of water. Wait five or ten minutes, and then decide if the snack is still as appealing as it was earlier.

- **Am I bored?** How many times do we mindlessly walk from a cabinet to the refrigerator and back to the cabinet looking for something to put into our mouth? Well, guess what? It's not the food that we need to be exciting—it is life at that moment that we wish were more exciting. Since we can't have that, we settle for the food. So the next time you mindlessly reach for something to put into your mouth, pull your hand back. Put on your shoes and go for a walk. Don't come back until you are no longer hungry. It will probably be 20 to 30 minutes.

- **Am I avoiding something?** When we don't want to face something that's bothering us or we're not ready to deal with it, we often turn to food for comfort or to fill a void. Problem at work? With family? Financial worries? Big or small, food will not solve your problems. You will have to deal with them even if you reach for that comfort food.

- **Am I eating out of want or need?** Let's say you're shopping and a pair of $600 shoes calls your name from across the aisle of the department store. You don't need them and really can't afford them, but they are stunning. You tell yourself that you're just going to try them on. They fit perfectly and make your legs look long and slim. Next thing you know, you're signing the credit card slip and taking those babies home, because you want them. Immediately. You give no thought to when you might wear them or how you're going to pay for them.

Food is the same. When you eat out of *want,* it is usually something your body doesn't need to lose weight. But when you eat out of *need,* you are eating because your body physically needs the food to survive. The differences are clear: You need to drink water, but you don't need to drink coffee. You need to eat protein, but you don't need a 10-ounce steak. When you eat out of need, you are eating the foods that supply nutrition, vitamins, and minerals to fuel your body. Anything else—ice cream, pizza, and tiramisu—is wanted, not needed.

- **How will it make me feel?** When you want to eat something that will derail your weight-loss efforts, do you consider how you will feel after you have consumed it? Train yourself to ask, "What am I going to feel like two hours from now after eating this cupcake or slice of pizza?" Most of the time it is never worth it. The cupcake isn't worth going off your diet, no matter whose birthday or party it is, or how good the treat looks. It is not worth the extra weight that you will need to lose. Knowing that you can have that cupcake on your Cheat Day encourages you to say no to your ongoing weight-loss efforts.

Cheat Days allow you to realize that on your six clean days you are eating out of need. On your Cheat Day, you are eating out of want. On your six clean days, you are fueling your body with nutritious foods to lose weight. When you eat out of need, you generally eat less. The reason you eat less is because you are eating balanced. You are satisfied. When you have fewer choices, you tend to also eat less out of boredom and have fewer cravings. In other words, the less you eat, the less you want.

Once you decide to begin a weight-loss program, you may find yourself thinking about food more than ever. Dealing with food restrictions can make you crave unhealthy foods. When you're told you can't have something, you want it even more. The fear of being hungry is a major setback for many people who want or need to lose weight, so recognizing the difference between physical and mental hunger is essential.

These two types of hunger may often feel the same, but there are some clues you should be aware of to be able to tell them apart. When your body needs fuel and energy, your brain sends you hunger signals. When it's physical, your hunger is gradual and isn't fixated on specific foods. This table shows you the different signs of mental and physical hunger.

Mental Hunger	Physical Hunger
Creates a need for something immediate	Results in low energy
Is triggered by cravings and emotions	Causes lightheadedness
Doesn't go away after eating	Takes a while to satisfy
Causes you to overeat	Goes away after you eat
Causes guilty feelings after eating	Leaves you feeling energized after eating

You may experience low energy or lightheadedness if it takes you a while to satisfy physical hunger. On the other hand, mental hunger is more sudden and urgent. It can be triggered by the craving for a certain food and usually involves absent-minded eating. It is also often paired with an upsetting emotion. Bad news or feeling anxious or depressed encourages you to want to eat something to make you feel better. Unlike physical hunger, mental hunger doesn't go away when you are full, causing you to overeat. It leaves you feeling guilty instead of energized and satisfied.

Recognizing mental hunger is the easy part; resisting it is the real battle. The first thing you should do when you're trying to determine if you're actually hungry or not is to stop and think about why you want to eat. Negative emotions can make you think you want to indulge in a slice of pizza or a serving of cake. Instead of immediately giving in, even if you're about to eat something healthy, reflect on your emotions and remind yourself that emotions can't make you hungry. They just convince you that you are. You should also pay attention to the time. When was the last time you ate? For example, if you just had a satisfying meal but you are looking for dessert, that's a *desire* for food—your body doesn't *need* it. You're just craving something sweet because you often have dessert and your body looks forward to it, whether you realize it or not. You can also try drinking a glass of water before deciding if you need a snack. Another way you can help yourself is to have healthy snacks on hand. Not only will you be able to satisfy your hunger with something good for you and your weight loss, but snacks that are high in protein and fiber will help keep hunger at bay.

Mental hunger is one of the biggest challenges when it comes to weight loss. Emotions are so closely tied to eating. We celebrate and grieve with food. Most social events and holidays seem to revolve around food. Cutting the ties with your cravings and emotional eating habits is hard and takes time, but it will happen. You're not just eating healthy food to lose weight; you're creating new habits for yourself without even realizing it.

. . . .

"Circumstances and situations do color life, but you have been given the mind to choose what the color will be."

—John Homer Miller

. . . .

THREE TYPES OF DAYS

Along with your Cheat Day, there are three types of days that you should be mindful of when it comes to weight loss: Weight-Loss Day, Maintain Day, and

Weight-Gain Day. You want to make sure if you are trying to lose weight that your six days are always Weight-Loss Days. You can do this by following your menu. The only time you should be incorporating a Maintain Day is if it's a holiday or vacation, and again that is up to each individual. You can go on vacation and have holidays and still lose weight. A Weight-Gain Day is not even an option. The only time a Weight-Gain Day will occur is when you are not prepared and have not planned your day well. A Weight-Gain Day rarely happens on purpose. In order to lose weight, you simply follow your program six days a week, and you will see the weight loss on the morning of the seventh day, your Cheat Day. Let's start by seeing examples of each day.

What Is a Weight-Loss Day?

A Weight-Loss Day is a day of eating on-program foods and following your menu 100 percent, from your first morning meal through your last snack in the evening. Along with eating clean, you have to eat less than your body needs to be in a constant state of restriction to lose weight. A *constant state of restriction* sounds much scarier than it is, but all it means is that you eat less food than your body and brain tell you they think they want. Once you understand what makes your day a Weight-Loss Day, it is important to stick to it six days a week.

It's entirely up to you to choose what time throughout the day you can eat your meals and snacks.

Typical Weight-Loss Day Menu

Breakfast: 4-egg-white omelet, with 1 cup vegetables. Spray a skillet pan with cooking spray (avocado or olive oil spray). Heat the skillet over medium heat. Whisk 4 egg whites until foamy and stir in 1 cup diced fresh vegetables, such as zucchini, onion, bell pepper, mushrooms, etc. Pour into the skillet and cook to desired doneness.

Snack: 1 medium apple, with 1 tablespoon peanut butter, apple butter, or nut butter. (While natural nut butters are best, they are not always available and can be expensive. Don't purchase reduced-fat nut butters—the good fats your body needs have been removed.)

. . . .

Lunch: Lettuce wraps of 6 thin slices turkey (about ¼ pound) and ½ cup bell peppers (fresh, jarred in vinegar, or roasted), rolled up in 2 large lettuce leaves. Or substitute ½ cup diced vegetables of your choosing for the peppers.

. . . .

Snack: 1 cup low-fat popcorn (100 calories, air popped or in a bag), such as Angie's BOOM-CHICKAPOP, or SkinnyPop, or Jollypop's 94-percent fat-free popcorn. Avoid flavored popcorns.

. . . .

Dinner: 6 ounces grilled chicken, with mustard dip (whisk together ¼ cup yellow mustard, 2 tablespoons white vinegar, 2 tablespoons water, ½ tablespoon olive oil, and 1 to 2 tablespoons hot sauce) and 2 cups steamed vegetables

. . . .

Snack: 15 nuts (almond, walnuts, pistachio, cashew, or mixed)

. . . .

What Is a Maintain Day?

A Maintain Day is when you eat more than you should to lose weight, but not enough to gain pounds. Your weight may fluctuate by a few pounds, but you end up staying around the same number. Many people don't lose weight because they will eat clean all day, but as soon as they get home, they eat whatever is in the pantry or refrigerator. Others may eat clean Monday through Thursday, but then cheat Friday, Saturday, and Sunday. What most people don't realize is they are really good maintainers. Even the healthiest eaters are maintainers because they simply eat too much healthy food to lose weight. Remember, at the end of the day you need to consume fewer calories than your body needs.

Typical Maintain Day Menu

Breakfast: 1 slice Ezekiel 4:9 bread, with 1 tablespoon peanut butter and banana slices

Lunch: 4-egg-white omelet, with 1 slice low-fat cheese and 1 cup steamed vegetables

Dinner: Green salad, shrimp scampi with mashed sweet potatoes and grilled vegetables

Snack: A few bites of chocolate cake

Snack: Bowl of fruit salad

Snack: 2 (6-ounce) glasses of wine

A Maintain Day is a day when you have more than a Weight-Loss Day, but not enough that you gain weight. You are giving your body what it needs to maintain your current weight.

Now that you can see the differences between a Weight-Loss Day, Maintain Day, and Weight-Gain Day, you can understand why the *Innovation Weight Loss*

Program works. You may recognize some things you have been doing that thwart your weight-loss efforts. If you have six Weight-Loss Days followed by a Cheat Day, you will lose weight. If you throw in a Maintain Day here and there, then it will take you two weeks to lose that same amount of weight. If you have three Weight-Loss Days followed by a Maintain Day, then another Weight-Loss Day and a Weight-Gain Day, and top it off with a Cheat Day, you won't lose weight. The more Maintain Days and Weight-Gain Days you allow yourself, the less likely the number on the scale will drop. In fact, if the Weight-Gain Days outnumber the Maintain Days, the numbers on the scale will go up.

What Is a Weight-Gain Day?

A Weight-Gain Day is a day when you eat more food and calories than your body needs to maintain its current weight. If you eat more food than your body needs to maintain your weight, then that food will be stored as fat and you will gain pounds.

A Weight-Gain Day is not a planned day like your Cheat Day. In order for the program to work, you get one day off each week, but this is not the same as a Weight-Gain Day. A Cheat Day is always planned and incorporated into your week—that is what makes it the Cheat Day. A Weight-Gain Day is *in addition* to your one day off and is not planned.

Typical Weight-Gain Day Menu

Breakfast: Cinnamon oatmeal with fruit and nuts

Snack: Bowl of fresh fruit salad

Lunch: Green salad topped with grilled chicken, avocado, toasted nuts, shredded cheese, and ranch dressing

Snack: 1 granola bar

Dinner: Chicken Parmesan and steamed broccoli

Snack: Package of M&M's

Snack: Apple, with 1 tablespoon peanut butter

It's not that every choice isn't a healthy choice here, but the combination of food makes this a Weight-Gain Day. Yes, you will see fruit salad on your *Innovation Weight Loss Program* menu as a snack, but it will be just a cup, not a big bowl. On a Weight-Gain Day, you can eat only unhealthy weight-gaining foods all day, or you may consume both healthy weight-loss and unhealthy weight-gaining foods.

RULE 2

ENJOY YOUR ONE CHEAT DAY EACH WEEK

Myth: You can't have your cake and lose weight too.

Truth: Oh yes—you can have your cake and lose weight too!

CHEAT DAY

A Cheat Day is the one day each week that you can eat the foods you denied yourself the other six days. You can have the brownie you craved on Wednesday or the Mudslide cocktail you passed up on Friday. With the Cheat Day, you get to enjoy all the foods you missed all week. Just think: You never again have to beat yourself up because you ate a bagel and an ice cream sundae, or a hamburger and a fully loaded baked potato while dieting. The funny thing is that once your Cheat Day arrives, you eventually won't choose the foods you've been thinking about all week! After several Cheat Days, you will discover which foods you really miss and will truly look forward to them. When it comes to handling Cheat Days, every person is different. Some people eat whatever they want all day, while others prefer to do so at one meal or just at dessert. Experiment and see what works best for you. There's no right or wrong way to enjoy your Cheat Day. At the end of a Cheat Day, you should feel like you've enjoyed what you've missed, but you're ready to start eating clean the next day. When your Cheat Day is used correctly, it helps you lose weight. How amazing is that?

For people who have tried multiple weight-loss diets, the idea of a Cheat Day seems unrealistic: How can I possibly eat whatever I want and still lose weight? What's interesting is that as your Cheat Day approaches, you'll eventually think differently about it. In the beginning, your Cheat Day can't come fast enough, and it's all you can think about. On your first few Cheat Days, you have a sense of guilt and think, am I really allowed to do this?

AM I DOING THE CHEAT DAY CORRECTLY?

As long as you eat whatever you want after your six days of clean eating, you are doing the Cheat Day correctly. That is what your Cheat Day is for. You can enjoy what you've been craving all week. Knowing that your Cheat Day is just a couple of days away will always give you a mental leg up when it comes to staying on program. Never eat just to eat, and focus on eating only what you missed and couldn't wait to have. It's okay to have healthy foods on your Cheat Day. The Cheat Day is designed so that you enjoy your cravings and the foods you missed, knowing you can have them if you want. You can incorporate cheat snacks with healthy meals or cheat meals with healthy snacks. Just make sure you are staying mindful and remember that the Cheat Day is not to eat from morning to night, or to choose foods you don't usually eat just to eat them. It's created to give you a day where you can eat whatever you want.

WON'T I RUIN EVERYTHING I WORKED SO HARD FOR ALL WEEK?

Absolutely not. In fact, if it weren't for your Cheat Day, you would probably give up halfway through the program. The Cheat Day saves you every week.

In the beginning, Cheat Days are all about eating all the foods you've missed all week. After a month or so, you'll find that you'll want to eat less on your Cheat Day. As your weight drops every week, your body and brain adjust to eating less. The foods you once thought you couldn't live without are no longer as appealing or as satisfying as the clean foods you eat the other six days a week.

Marcy, a client who loves food, told me that when she woke up in the past, the first thing she'd think about was what she would eat that day. For breakfast, Marcy loved spicy tacos with eggs and turkey sausage. When we planned her program, she realized she could include these foods on her Cheat Day. She loved her Cheat Day! In the beginning she told me about everything she ate and drank, including the many times that she'd felt nauseous and bloated from overeating. After a couple of weeks on program, she noticed that she was eating less and less on her Cheat Day. Not because she wanted to, but because she was filling up so much faster. By the time she was finished with breakfast on her Cheat Days, she was too full to enjoy other foods she thought she had missed. "It makes me so sad that I don't want to eat everything I can on my Cheat Day anymore." When I told her that she could, she answered, "No, I tried!" The more weight she lost, the less interested Marcy became in her Cheat Day foods. She said she now thought about everything she was going to eat on her Cheat Day and planned it out so she could fit in what she really wanted.

During the first few Cheat Days, you will feel like you miss everything in sight. Foods you never even knew you liked become something you crave. After you abuse it, you will realize that you need to put a little work into the Cheat Day and think about what foods you really do miss. What are the foods you used to wish you could have when you were trying to diet 24/7? Is there anything specific? Anything worth waiting for? Most of the time we think we want things until we have permission to have them. Then we realize we never wanted them at all. Such was the case with Adam's and Eve's forbidden fruit. You want what you can't have. If someone says it is off limits, it is all you think about.

Janet, another client, likes to go food shopping for her Cheat Day. She said it feels liberating to take her cart through the grocery store aisles and buy the foods that she always wanted to eat but never allowed herself. When Janet first started the program and went shopping for her Cheat Day, her cart was filled with chips and cookies. On her Cheat Days, she would graze all day long on her purchases. By 11 p.m., she would try to squeeze in whatever junk food she could before going to bed. As a result, she felt horrible all night and even worse the next morning. For Janet, it only took her three overstuffed Cheat Days until she promised herself that she would never do that again. Janet reminded herself that she didn't have to eat everything in just one Cheat Day. Another one was just a week away.

It only takes a few Cheat Days for your mind to catch up to your body. Focus on the foods you miss and your choices will satisfy you.

Think about the foods that excite you and make you happy. What if you picked one meal? Breakfast? Lunch? Dinner? Brunch? What would each meal include? What kind of dessert would make you happy? A slice of pie or cake? An ice cream sundae? Chocolate mousse? Once you figure out what foods excite you, it becomes easier to plan your Cheat Day. You learn which foods you crave and which ones you can do without, because you can have them on another Cheat Day.

Tara is a healthy eater and keeps her diet clean six days a week. She never strays. She lost 40 pounds from her five-foot frame and now weighs a healthy 94 pounds. She looks and feels amazing. What does Tara have on her Cheat Day? It is the same Cheat Day every week. She eats clean for breakfast and lunch. Then dinner is always what I call a *candy salad*: a big green salad tossed with dried cranberries, nuts, avocado, cheese, grilled chicken or fish, apples, and candied pecans. Sometimes she adds corn, sour cream, and salsa, and tops it with a balsamic vinaigrette or creamy ranch dressing. Later in the evening, Tara indulges in a couple of scoops of ice cream topped with chocolate sauce and whipped cream while watching TV. Why not enjoy other treats? I mean, it's her Cheat Day after all. The answer is simple. Tara has already been down that road. She tried eating other things—French fries and burgers—on her Cheat Days, thinking she would still eat her ice cream when she got home. But what happened was quite the opposite. After she ate those other things during the day, she was so full and bloated that she couldn't enjoy her ice cream at night.

For Tara, just because she could eat more didn't mean she wanted to. She found it more satisfying to stick to the foods that she knew she would enjoy.

SNOWBALL EFFECT: THE ALL-OR-NOTHING PERSON

The Cheat Day is an amazing tool, especially for the all-or-nothing person. These are people who, once they start something, cannot stop doing it. Whether they are hungry or not, it doesn't matter. Once they have gone off their diets, they just keep going, knowing that they will have to start over again. They eat everything they possibly can before that day arrives. For some, it can last a week or even a month. This is what I call the *snowball effect*. It starts small, but by the time they are done rolling down that hill, their snowball is as big as a mountain—with the pounds to prove it. What most people do not realize is that only happens when those foods are off-limits.

If you're an all-or-nothing person and your nutrition program does not include unhealthy-food choices, you probably tend to binge uncontrollably. Now, with the Cheat Day in your program, you can have those foods once a week. Whatever foods you would normally go for are in reach at all times. Now that you can have them, guess what happens? I'll bet you already know the answer. You won't look for them. All of a sudden, when they are *allowed* and you have *permission* to eat them, you'll no longer want them. They won't be as desirable. Yes, you may still have them once or twice, but then suddenly, you're over them.

Kami could not get over the fact that she could start her Cheat Day with a bagel. She said she had not eaten a bagel in seven years. The funny thing is that after her third Cheat Day, she no longer wanted a bagel. She soon preferred eating the same protein bar on her Cheat Days that she ate on her clean days. Would she have felt like that if her first few Cheat Days didn't include the bagel? Absolutely not. She would have wanted that bagel every Sunday when her family was having them. Another important thing to point out about Kami is that she didn't eat a bagel in seven years, but she still had a weight problem—until she started the *Innovation Weight Loss Program*. Sometimes, just because we avoid eating foods that we think are unhealthy doesn't mean we are going to lose weight.

Mentally, when we are given permission, it can sometimes change the course of our actions. In return, we do the right thing instead of continually sabotaging ourselves with the wrong things. Since starting the *Innovation Weight Loss Program*, Kami has lost a total of 42 pounds and has maintained her goal weight for more than five years. She still tells me that she never eats her bagel. While she definitely enjoys her Cheat Day with other favorite foods, bagels are no longer part of her must-have foods.

The problem today with most diets is that they are not realistic. Some want you to give up everything you love, and others want you to include little things that tease you. It is not realistic for an all-or-nothing person, which 90 percent of food addicts are, to have a little piece of pie and then move on to clean and healthy foods. A piece of anything is not a reward for a food addict. It is a tease that will completely throw that person off the rails.

You have to understand that you cannot expect to live forever without foods you love—just like you cannot eliminate a food group. You cannot live without carbs—and why would you want to? Sure, you will lose weight faster, but you will put on twice as much when you start eating them again. The only way to create weight loss for a lifetime and a healthy way of eating is to create a balance that works for you. Since 90 percent of the population is in the all-or-nothing category, the Cheat Day relates to them and works for them. The Cheat Day also works for the average social person who has that big event or a weekly party night out. For the other 10 percent who may not be all-or-nothing food types, the Cheat Day works for them because they use it to incorporate eating whatever they want into their busy lives. There is always a day in the week for them when they either *want* or *need* to go off their healthy clean eating. The Cheat Day is that day for everyone who wants it.

WON'T I GAIN WEIGHT ON MY CHEAT DAY?

While it's hard to believe, you will lose more weight over a period of time with a once-a-week Cheat Day. There are a few reasons to support this. The first is that you would most likely go off program if you didn't have the Cheat Day. The Cheat Day keeps you on and in control of the six weight-loss days, and that is what you need to lose weight. Without the Cheat Day, you wouldn't have the same control and you would find yourself going off program altogether.

Another reason the Cheat Day makes you lose more weight is that you confuse your body with the extra food and unhealthier choices each week. On your Cheat Day, you take in all the extra food choices that you wouldn't have on your six clean days. So the day after the Cheat Day, when you once again eat clean and on program, your body thinks you are starting a new diet. All of a sudden, it has to work harder in order to keep up with less food from the day before. In return, it will start using the stored fat that you have on your body because you are giving it less food.

So the Cheat Day shakes things up. It makes your body believe that you are starting a new weight-loss program every week. The Cheat Day interrupts the cycle so your body doesn't get used to what you give it every week. The average dieter loses more weight in the first week than in the remainder of the program. The reason for this outcome is that the body isn't used to what it's been given and has to work harder to keep up. The Cheat Day not only confuses the body; it also makes sure that it doesn't get used to the same foods every week. When you have your Cheat Day, it instantly makes your body start working harder to understand and keep up with what is being taken in. Every week you will get weight-loss results because your body thinks it is starting a new program.

Fake Weight

What also happens after a Cheat Day is that you gain water/fluid weight from consuming extra food. That's why weight fluctuates so often, mostly due to extra salt, fluid, and calorie intake that the body hasn't fully processed yet. You don't gain *fat weight* from one day. Think of it like this: You have trillions of fat cells in your body. Your objective is to shrink your fat cells. You do that by eating on program six days a week. Fat cells don't shrink overnight, but they also don't grow overnight. It would take more than one Cheat Day for new fat cells to grow. However, you have to be careful because if you don't go right back on program after your Cheat Day, then you will be adding Cheat Day on top of Cheat Day—and that's how fat cells grow. If you go right back on program after your Cheat Day, then you will get rid of the extra water and fluid immediately, and your body will start the process of losing weight again and go back to the process of shrinking old fat cells. However, if you do another cheat (even just one bite of something), then you will not lose that extra weight and your body will go into a Maintain Day. A Maintain Day is having more than what is on program, but not enough to consider a cheat—for example, having extra on-program snacks or bigger portions. The best way to avoid any weight gain or Maintain Days is to go right back on program after a Cheat Day. As soon as you go right back on program, you will start losing weight. Bottom line: It's important that you get right back on program the day after a Cheat Day. If you do, you will lose the *fake weight* and start losing *real fat* again.

When the Scale Goes Up after a Cheat Day

Of course, when you have a Cheat Day and eat more, the number on the scale will temporarily go up. Don't weigh yourself the night of or the day after a Cheat Day. Seeing the number go up can cause you to mentally sabotage yourself—and that number can send you on an eating frenzy. Remember, when we are trying to lose weight, we don't need an excuse to go off program. A higher number on the scale may be all it takes for you to abandon the program. So I am forewarning you that the scale is going to be higher the night of your Cheat Day and the day after the Cheat Day. There is nothing you can do about it because it's fake weight, and it will go back down once you start eating clean again. The best way to handle the scale is to not go on it after a Cheat Day. Follow the program, and more importantly, trust the program. Weigh yourself the morning of every Cheat Day. If you do this, the number will be lower each subsequent Cheat Day morning.

RULE 3

AFTER YOUR CHEAT DAY, GO RIGHT BACK ON PROGRAM

Myth: I won't be able to get back on program after a Cheat Day.

Truth: Just like you craved Cheat Day foods, you'll find that you can't wait to get right back to six days of clean eating.

Ninety-nine percent of my clients can't wait to start eating clean again after a Cheat Day. After feeling so good, so much lighter and thinner all week, you'll have your Cheat Day and suddenly feel bloated and heavy, normal but uncomfortable. By the night of your Cheat Day, you'll find yourself thinking, "I can't wait to eat clean again and feel lighter and thinner." One of the reasons you will be so eager to get right back on program is that you will want that lighter, thinner feeling back. One of the most exciting things about the program is that once you start following your menu, it only takes a couple of days until you feel that you are in control. You won't mind going to bed a little hungry. When you wake up, you'll look forward to getting dressed because you won't be busting out of your clothes. Well, the day after the Cheat Day, you are going to want that feeling back. Remember, you will feel that thinner feeling all week long, up until your Cheat Day. Then all of a sudden it is replaced with indulgences that you thought you wanted more than anything. After a day of eating whatever you want, you realize that what you want more than anything is to have that light, thinner feeling back.

Anyone who has tried to lose weight knows the feeling once a few pounds are lost. First, your face looks thinner, your love handles are smaller, or your arms feel lighter. On the *Innovation Weight Loss Program*, you will feel lighter and thinner as each week passes. I tell my clients that they may be behind on their bills or having trouble at work, but if their pants zip up easily, then everything is right in their world.

DON'T JUST DO THE PROGRAM–LIVE THE PROGRAM

Eventually the *Innovation Weight Loss Program* will be a part of your daily life, like brushing your teeth. Eating six days on program followed by one Cheat Day is something that you will be able to do forever. You fuel your body six days a week, then you enjoy and indulge one day. Sometimes when we just do a program, we focus more on being done with it so we can go back to our old ways. There is no *over* or *end* with this program. This is a way of life that you'll come to love.

Choose Your Hard

Some days it will be hard to go back on program after a Cheat Day. You might want to physically, but mentally your mind is challenging your body. This is when you need to *choose your hard*. Is it harder to start a weight-loss program when you have so much going on, or is it harder to deal with all the things you have going on when you feel uncomfortable, unhappy, and overweight? Is it harder to eat on program and walk away from a table full of temptation, or is it harder to see the numbers rise on the scale? When you think about what will ultimately make you happy, it becomes easier to choose your hard.

If You Struggle to Get Back on Program

If you find that you have a week when you are struggling to get back on program, here are some tips to help you:

- **Small goals lead to big goals:** When you need a little motivation, think about what your big goal is. You want to lose 10, 20, or 50 pounds? If you have a number in your head, that is your big goal. Now it is necessary to make little goals to get you to your big goal. For example, "I am going to lose one pound every week for a total of four pounds this month," or "I am going to lose 10 pounds by Memorial Day, which is in six weeks." Wherever you are right now, think about the little goals that will get you to your ultimate goal.

- **Embrace the hunger:** If you are feeling a little hungry, know that it's okay. You are eating less than you used to, so it's natural to feel hungrier when you cut back on the amount of food you consume. Use your hunger as a tool for reaching your ultimate weight-loss goal. When you feel those hunger pangs, it means that the *Innovation Weight Loss Program* is working for you and you are losing weight. Also know that those feelings of hunger will disappear in 10 to 20 minutes if you're not truly hungry.

- **Positive thoughts and positive actions give positive results:** Thinking positively about what you want and what is important to you is a game changer when it comes to weight loss. When you are happy and positive, you will make happy and positive choices, which will give you positive results. Remember that your mind is the most powerful organ in your entire body. It can heal you and it can make you sick. If you want to feel good, healthy, and stay on program, you have to constantly remind yourself that is what you want. You must believe that you can do it, and you have to follow through every day with how you feel.

- **Plan and be prepared for your days and week:** I can't say it enough—if you plan your days and your food, you will have the best results. If you let yourself wing it and try to get through the day without a plan, you are going to find yourself at a point with nothing to eat or unable to find what you need. When you get to that hungry-starving feeling, you will end up grabbing anything in sight—whether it's on program or not. When you plan, you don't ever have to worry about getting to such an uncomfortable level.

- **Make a choice:** At the end of the day, it's always a choice. Is this something you really want? Then you have to really work for it. If you know that losing weight will make you feel better, look better, and just overall be happier, then you need to do it. Sometimes it's about more than just us. When you are happy, everyone around you is happy; but when you are not happy, you are affecting everyone around you as well. If you find that you need to change and become the person you always wanted to be— the person who has lost weight and feels great—then you have to follow your program. Make the choice to stay on program, working hard on the challenging days and enjoying the days that come easier.

. . . .

"Show the world who you are, not by what you say, but what you do."

—Unknown

. . . .

RULE 4

LISTEN TO YOUR MIND AND BODY

. . . .

Myth: I can only lose weight if I don't eat carbs.

Reality: You will lose weight only if you include a balance of healthy carbs and protein.

. . . .

On the *Innovation Weight Loss Program*, you don't give up any food groups to lose weight. Your body needs healthy proteins, fats, and carbs to function properly. You cannot live without them. Diets that omit any of these can be unhealthy and even dangerous.

PROTEIN IS IMPORTANT TO YOUR DIET

Every cell in the body contains proteins. Consuming protein is essential to help your body repair cells and make new ones. While all meat, poultry, seafood, beans and peas, eggs, processed soy products, nuts, and seeds contain protein, it doesn't mean they are good for you or will help you lose weight.

Below are examples of healthy weight-loss proteins and some approximate serving sizes.

Protein Choices for Women

- 4 to 6 ounces cooked turkey, chicken, or fish
- ½ cup cooked beans, such as white, black, kidney

- 4 egg whites (¾ cup liquid egg whites) or 1 large whole egg
- 2 ounces nonfat or low-fat cheese
- 1 cup cooked quinoa
- ¾ cup plain nonfat Greek yogurt

Protein Snacks for Women

- ¼ cup nuts
- 1 tablespoon peanut butter, almond butter, or mixed-nut butter
- 1 slice nonfat or low-fat cheese

Protein Choices for Men

- 8 to 10 ounces turkey, chicken, fish, or steak (filet mignon or London broil)
- 1 cup cooked beans or legumes
- 8 to 10 egg whites (1½ cups liquid egg whites) or 2 whole eggs
- 3 to 4 slices nonfat or low-fat cheese
- 2 cups cooked quinoa

> ## Protein Snacks for Men
>
> - ¼ cup nuts
> - 2 tablespoons peanut butter, almond butter, or mixed-nut butter
> - 2 slices nonfat or low-fat cheese
> - 1 cup plain nonfat Greek yogurt

Certain Fats Are Important to Your Diet

Most people who come to me for help with weight-loss issues are confused about fats. Too often, they believe that if they could eliminate fats from their diets, their weight problems would be solved. Nothing could be further from the truth. Healthy fats are important because they provide essential fatty acids, keep skin soft, deliver fat-soluble vitamins, aid in weight loss, and provide fuel. Since it's easy to get confused about good fats vs. bad fats, here's an explanation of the fats you can enjoy and those to avoid.

Fats to Eat in Moderation

Unsaturated fats are the healthy fats you want to seek out. They include polyunsaturated fatty acids and monounsaturated fats. Both monounsaturated and polyunsaturated fats—when eaten in moderation—

can help lower cholesterol levels, reduce the risk of heart disease, and help with weight loss.

Polyunsaturated fats, found mostly in vegetable oils, help lower both blood cholesterol levels and triglyceride levels, especially when they are used in place of saturated fats. One type of polyunsaturated fat is omega-3 fatty acids, whose potential heart-healthy boosters are found in fatty fish (salmon, trout, catfish, mackerel), flaxseed meal, and walnuts. Fish contain the most effective omega-3s.

The other *good fat* unsaturated fats are monounsaturated fats, thought to reduce the risk of heart disease. Mediterranean countries consume lots of these fats—primarily in the form of olive oil. This dietary component is credited with the low levels of heart disease in residents of the Mediterranean region. These heart-healthy fats are also typically a good source of the antioxidant vitamin E, a nutrient often lacking in American diets. They can be found in olives, avocados, hazelnuts, almonds, Brazil nuts, cashews, sesame seeds, pumpkin seeds, and olive, canola, and peanut oils.

Fats to Avoid

Saturated and trans fats are the two types of fats that should be eaten sparingly or avoided altogether. Both can raise cholesterol levels and increase the risk for heart disease. These fats contribute to the world's obesity epidemic.

The fat molecules in saturated fats have no double bonds between their carbon molecules because they are saturated with hydrogen molecules. Saturated fats include meat, butter, lard, poultry skin, cream, full-fat cheese, and whole-fat milk products. They are also found in coconut oil and palm oil.

There are two types of trans fats, also known as trans-unsaturated fatty acids. One kind occurs naturally in small amounts in dairy products and meat, which are of minor concern, especially if you eat low-fat dairy products and lean meats. The second type of trans fats are industrially produced from vegetable fats and then hardened into partially hydrogenated fats. They're used extensively in fast-food frying, processed baked goods and snacks, vegetable shortening, and some margarines.

Fats to Eat and Fats to Avoid

Most foods contain a combination of various fats but are classified according to the dominant one. This chart lists sources of the good-for-you unsaturated fats as well as some examples of fats you'll want to avoid.

Avoid Saturated Fats and Trans Fats	Eat in Moderation Polyunsaturated Fats	Incorporate Monounsaturated Fats
Butter	Corn oil	Canola oil
Lard	Fish oils	Almond oil
Meat, lunch meat	Soybean oil	Walnut oil
Poultry, poultry skin	Safflower oil	Olives, olive oil
Coconut products	Sesame oil	Peanut oil
Palm oil, palm kernel oil, and their products	Cottonseed oil	Avocados, avocado oil
Dairy foods (other than reduced fat)	Sunflower oil	Nuts, seeds
Partially hydrogenated oils		Peanut butter, almond butter, mixed-nut butters

Carbs Are Important to Your Diet

In nutrition, carbohydrate—carb for short—refers to the third macronutrient (the other two are protein and fat). This is why it's so important to have a balanced meal or snack that consists of healthy proteins, fats, and carbs. Consuming all three in proper amounts guarantees that your body is properly fueled. Dietary carbs can be split into three main categories:

- **Sugars:** Sweet, short-chain carbohydrates found in foods; examples are glucose, fructose, galactose, and sucrose

- **Starches:** Long chains of glucose molecules, which eventually get broken down into glucose in the digestive system

- **Fiber:** Indigestible material in food, some of which can be used by the bacteria in the digestive system

Stored Energy = Weight Gain

The main purpose of eating foods that contain carbohydrates is to provide energy for your body. Most carbs get broken down or transformed into glucose, which can be used as energy. Carbs can also be turned into fat, which is what you want to avoid.

When you eat too many carbohydrates, they are stored for later use. Stored energy turns into fat. The only time stored energy doesn't turn into fat is if you need it to run a marathon or participate in a triathlon. If you're not a competitive athlete or training to become one, then there's no reason to overeat carbs and store energy because you won't lose weight. Exactly the opposite will occur. You will gain weight because fat will be stored.

When you eat on program, you will not store energy because you will not be overeating. In fact, you will be eating less than your body currently needs (remember, you should be a little hungry), and your body will use stored fat cells to run properly. When you eat less but keep your meals balanced by staying on program, you will actually use the stored fat your body has and lose weight.

When you take in less than your body currently needs, you will feel a little hungry, but this forces the body to use the stored fat, which is how we lose weight. However, this can only be accomplished when you are following your balanced program.

Healthy Carbs

Fruits and vegetables supply healthy carbs to your diet. They keep your diet balanced because they work with protein to provide a balanced day of feeding muscles while providing energy to cells. Of course, eating too much of healthy foods is not good for weight loss either. So make sure when you enjoy fruits and vegetables that you only have the portion that is allowed on your menu. Here are the vegetables and fruits that are on program:

Vegetables	Fruits
Arugula	Apple
Asparagus	Avocado (1/2)
Bok choy	Banana
Broccoli	Berries (all) (1 cup)
Brussel sprouts	Cantaloupe (1 cup)
Cabbage	Cherries (1 cup)
Cauliflower	Grapes (1 cup)
Celery	Melon (all) (1 cup)
Cucumber	Nectarine
Green beans	Orange
Kale	Papaya
Leeks	Peach
Lettuce (all)	Pear
Mushrooms	Pineapple (1 cup)
Onions	
Peppers (red, green, yellow)	
Peas	
Radishes	
Spinach	

One of the reasons I studied nutrition was that my father was a diabetic. When I was 16, he had to have one of his legs amputated. I was in the room with him after the surgery, and everyone was coming to see him and bringing him gifts (food, of course). Someone brought a bowl of grapes. He loves grapes and started eating them. Before we knew it, all the machines were sending out alarm signals—and the nurses and doctor came running in. They had to give him an insulin shot. We all were stunned. Just because he had eaten grapes, his insulin levels had gone off the charts. Seeing how frightened I was, the doctor explained to me that the body can't tell one kind of sugar from another. Sugar is sugar, whether it's natural sugar in fruit or processed sugar in candy bars. So I asked, "Why not eat candy instead of fruit if it's all the same?" He explained, "With fruit you are eating carbs that convert to sugar, but you are also getting fiber and vitamins. With candy, you only get carbs and unhealthy fats." I then understood that if you eat too much of any sugar or carb, the excess is stored as body fat. At the end of the day it always comes down to choices. This makes me think of a quote I once read that went something like this: "Every morning we get 24 golden hours that are free of charge. For some, they are cut way too short. If you have your 24 golden hours, then treat them as a gift—one you'll want to fill with health, happiness, and the very best choices you can make for yourself and those you love."

Fiber Is Important to Your Diet

Dietary fiber is the roughage or indigestible portions of plant-based foods, including fruits, vegetables, nuts, beans, and whole grains. While fiber doesn't provide energy directly, it does feed the friendly bacteria in the digestive system. Fiber can lower blood sugar, cut cholesterol, may even prevent colon cancer, and help you avoid hemorrhoids.

Fiber comes in two varieties, both of which are beneficial to health:

- Soluble fiber, which dissolves in water, can help lower glucose levels and help lower blood cholesterol

- Insoluble fiber, which does not dissolve in water, can help food move through your digestive system, promoting regularity and helping prevent constipation

The best high-fiber foods that are on program include: avocado, almonds, apples, broccoli, Brussels sprouts, chia seeds, cucumbers, edamame, peas, pear, raspberries, and whole wheat bread.

RULE 5

EXERCISE TO HELP YOU LOSE WEIGHT AND FEEL GREAT

. . . .

Myth: I can't lose weight because I can't exercise.

Reality: You don't need to exercise to lose weight.

. . . .

Should I exercise? Do I need to? I hate it. It makes me hungry! Whether you want to exercise or not has less to do with having to. Exercise is good for you. There are many reasons you should exercise, but when it comes to weight loss, it's about a *want* not a *need*.

Q: Do I need to exercise to lose weight?

A: No.

Reason: The scale is all about what you are eating. If you eat on program, you will lose weight whether you exercise or not.

Ellen was a client who came in and physically could not exercise. She had slipped discs in her spine and painful knees. To look at her, she just looked overweight and frumpy. The weight made her 58-year-old body look like she was 70. I asked about less-strenuous exercises, such as swimming or walking, but they were not an option for her. Her doctor had said no exercise. I explained that if she ate on program and followed her menu, then she would not have to worry about working out or exercising. So she started her program. In six months, she had lost 40 pounds. She looked amazing.

Even more important, she felt great. Her 58-year-old body now looks ten years younger!

Q: Can I exercise, not eat healthy, and lose weight?

A: No.

Most people eat more because they exercise. When you exercise, you feel that you are entitled to eat more because you exercised. Unfortunately, it doesn't work like that. Exercise has to be *in addition to* your weight-loss program. Therefore, you don't add more food because you exercise. What you do need to add is extra water. When working out, you should be drinking at least half your body weight in ounces of water a day.

When 39-year-old Trina came to me three years ago, she couldn't understand why she couldn't lose a pound because she had been working out three hours a day. I explained to her that she had to eat less and exercise less if she wanted to see her muscles emerge from the fat on her body. Trina couldn't understand how that was possible until I explained that she already had tried it her way, and it clearly wasn't working—let's try it my way. I set her up with a menu. She was allowed to exercise just one hour every day. Trina could not believe how quickly she was losing weight and how long and lean she now looked. She realized she was eating so much more food than she thought, and a lot of it had to do with the exercise. It was making her so hungry that she would often eat whatever she could get her hands on. Now Trina stays on program with her six days of healthy eating followed by her Cheat Day, and she exercises for one hour daily. She is 20 pounds lighter!

Q: Will I gain weight if I exercise with weights?

A: No.

Muscle does not weigh more than fat and fat does not weigh more than muscle. A pound is a pound whether it's fat, muscle, water, or feathers. But because muscle is dense, it looks better than fat. When you replace fat with muscle, you may weigh the same, but you will look trimmer.

Q: Why should I work out if it's not going to help me lose weight?

A: Exercise helps you lose weight if you are eating on program.

Exercise is most beneficial when you eat on program and take in healthy portions of foods that are designed to help you lose weight. While it's important to exercise in addition to eating on program for weight loss, it's also good for other health reasons too. Exercise is good for your heart and lungs. Even naturally thin people who don't exercise have heart problems and breathing issues that can be improved with exercise. While weight loss is important, total health is more important because it doesn't matter how thin you are if you are sick.

Bones: Bone is living tissue that responds to exercise by becoming stronger, especially as we age. Exercising allows us to maintain muscle strength, coordination, and balance, which in turn help to prevent falls and related fractures.

Muscles: Muscle strength declines as people age, but studies report that when people exercise they are stronger and leaner than others in their age group. If you don't use your muscles, you will lose them.

You look better! That's right, you appear thinner when you exercise. Muscle is more dense than fat. Picture fat: It's loose, flabby, and takes up space. You look bigger when you are what I like to call *skinny fat,* someone who loses weight but doesn't work out. When you work out and lose weight, you are thin and fit. The muscles of your body become denser and take up less room than fat, making you appear smaller and tighter.

Getting Started with Exercise

Before you start any exercise program, get a physical from your doctor or other health care professional. Some people can't work out; if that's you, then follow your medical orders.

Okay, you received the go-ahead to start exercising, but you don't know where to begin. Here are some ways to get started:

- **Walk:** It's easy, available, and costs nothing. Brisk walking provides great cardiovascular exercise and helps lower levels of LDL (bad) cholesterol while increasing levels of HDL (good) cholesterol. The American Stroke Association says that a brisk 30-minute walk every day helps prevent and control the high blood pressure that causes strokes. It's one of the easiest and most effective things you can do for your body, both mentally and physically. Get a walking buddy or join a walking group.

- **Join a gym:** Many gyms offer introductory sessions with trainers who show you how to use free weights and machines. You can also take exercise classes, if offered.

- **Hire a trainer:** Personal trainers train you one-on-one or in a group. Go to your local YMCA or other gym, or find a trainer who will come to your home. A quality trainer doesn't need much space or equipment to create a program for you. Personal trainers are great because they can make sure you are working to your ability while maintaining proper form. Many will offer once-a-month training where you can do the exercises they show you on your own for the entire month, so it's much less expensive. Then you can go back and get new exercises for the next month.

- **Yoga:** Downward dogs and sun salutations do more than just burn calories and tone muscles. Yoga is a total mind-body workout that combines strengthening and stretching poses with deep breathing and meditation. Yoga is especially good for people with limitations and injuries. You can do it at your local gym or yoga studio, or hire a one-on-one yoga instructor to come to your home.

- **Pilates:** If you are looking to strengthen your back and abs, then Pilates is the way to go. You will gain long, lean muscles and improve flexibility, which helps prevent injuries. Learn a couple of moves and you can do them every day.

- **Run:** One of my favorite forms of exercise is running. Put on a pair of sneakers and you can go right out your front door. If you are just beginning and a little hesitant on how to begin, there are many smartphone apps to choose from to help you get started.

- **Swim:** A great exercise for everyone is swimming. As long as you know how to do it, the benefits are many. It improves muscle definition and strength, builds bone mass, burns calories, and reduces inflammation. And if you are looking for an exercise that improves heart and lung capacity but is gentle on your joints, swimming is a top choice.

- **Cycle:** Something that was once only for outdoors is now one of the most popular indoor exercise classes. And if you can't make it to the gym and can't ride outdoors, you can purchase an indoor bike and cycle right at home. Cycling is a great exercise that targets both cardiovascular and endurance-improving heart health and lung capacity.

There are many options to start or improve your exercise routine. The choices are endless, and so is the potential for success.

RULE 6

FOLLOW ONE OF THE INNOVATION PROGRAM WEIGHT-LOSS MENUS

Below are two basic weight-loss menus—follow either menu and you will lose weight. The most important thing to remember is that the closer you follow the menu, the more weight you will lose.

MENU 1 (WOMEN)

In addition to the meals and snacks outlined below, all *Innovation Weight Loss Program* meals and snacks are the right portions to keep you on your plan. Find a complete list in our Food Store at innovationweight loss.com.

Start your day with 8 to 12 ounces hot or warm water and a lemon wedge. Drink 12 ounces of water before each meal.

Breakfast (Choose One)

- 1 slice whole wheat, Ezekiel 4:9, or Arnold's low-calorie bread, with 1 tablespoon peanut butter or almond butter, topped with ½ sliced banana

- Power Crunch Original Protein Bar
- 4-egg-white omelet or scrambled egg whites, with 1 cup steamed vegetables (see list under Rule 4, Healthy Carbs)
- 5 to 6 ounces nonfat Greek yogurt (any flavor), with ½ cup plain Cheerios or ½ cup of any berries mixed in
- Innovation breakfast meal (order online at innovationweightloss.com)

Lunch (Choose One)

- 4 ounces grilled chicken, seafood, or turkey, with 1 cup chopped lettuce and 1 cup vegetables (see list under Rule 4, Healthy Carbs)
- Vegetarian salad of 1 cup chopped lettuce and 1 cup vegetables, topped with 2 tablespoons nuts or one of the following:
  - 1 ounce (¼ cup shredded or 2 slices) light or low-fat cheese
  - ¼ cup chickpeas
  - ¼ cup canned hearts of palm, drained
  - ¼ cup steamed edamame

- ◻ 1 hard-boiled egg
- ◻ ¼ avocado
- 6 slices low-sodium turkey or chicken, rolled with 2 slices light or low-fat cheese
- 5 ounces light tuna salad or light chicken salad (purchase light or low-fat chicken salad, or add 1 tablespoon light mayonnaise to water-packed tuna)
- Innovation lunch meal (order online at innovationweightloss.com)

Dinner (Choose One)

- 6 ounces skinless grilled or rotisserie chicken or turkey
- 2 cups zucchini linguini and ¼ cup light or low-fat cheese or 2 tablespoons grated Parmesan cheese, with optional lemon and 1 tablespoon olive oil and seasonings (see list at the end of rule 6, On-Program Fats, Herbs, and Spices)
- 6 ounces any baked or broiled fish or shellfish
- Innovation dinner meal (order online at innovationweightloss.com)

Every day you can have up to an additional 2 cups steamed or roasted vegetables (see list under Rule 4, Healthy Carbs) as a side with lunch or dinner.

Dressing for salad: 1 tablespoon oil and unlimited red wine vinegar, white vinegar, or apple cider vinegar, and any spices from the list at the end of rule 6, On-Program Fats, Herbs, and Spices.

No sauces, gravy, butter, soy sauce, breadcrumbs/breading, or dressing (other than as described above) of any kind.

Everything can be cooked and/or ordered with any seasoning from list at the end of rule 6, On-Program Fats, Herbs, and Spices.

Snacks

The program allows three snacks per day, one from each category. If you don't want a snack from category 3, you can have a second snack from category 1 or 2, but never more than one snack from category 3. Snacks can be eaten in any order and at any point during the day or evening. You do not have to eat all or any of your snacks. Eat what you need. Less is best when trying to lose weight.

Category 1 (Choose One)

- 1 cup cut-up fruit or 1 piece of fruit

Category 2 (Choose One)

- 3 cups regular or sea salt, low-fat popcorn
- Iced coffee or latte with nonfat milk
- 1 cup any flavor Cheerios (dry)
- 1 cup steamed or raw vegetables, with ¼ cup hummus
- Apple, with 1 tablespoon peanut butter or almond butter
- 1 small avocado, with drizzle of lemon or lime juice

Category 3 (Choose One)

- Innovation snack
- 4 ounces wine or 1 ounce alcohol
- ¼ cup nuts
- 4- to 5-ounce snack pack ready-made, fat-free chocolate or vanilla pudding, or

½ cup fat-free chocolate or vanilla instant box pudding with 2 tablespoons whipped cream or Cool Whip

- 2 whole wheat crackers, with 1 ounce light or low-fat cheese

Drinks

- Unlimited water

- Coffee and tea (no sugar, but you can use artificial sweetener and splash of skim milk)

- Diet drinks permitted

MENU 2 (MEN)

(This menu also can be used by women who want to lose 40 or more pounds.)

In addition to the meals and snacks outlined below, all Innovation meals and snacks are the right portions to keep you on your plan. Find a complete list in our Food Store at innovationweightloss.com.

Start your day with 12 ounces hot or warm water and a lemon wedge. Drink 12 ounces of water before each meal.

Breakfast (Choose One)

- 6- to 8-egg-white omelet, with 1 cup vegetables (see list under Rule 4, Healthy Carbs)

- 1 cup Cheerios Protein, with ½ cup skim or unsweetened almond milk

- Power Crunch Original Protein Bar, with 1 cup cut-up fruit or 1 piece of fruit

- 2 slices low-calorie whole wheat or rye toast, with 1 tablespoon peanut butter and small sliced banana

- Innovation breakfast meal (order online at innovationweightloss.com)

Lunch (Choose One)

- 6 ounces chicken, turkey, quinoa, or vegetable burger

- 6 ounces grilled chicken, fish, or turkey, with 2 cups steamed or grilled vegetables (see list under Rule 4, Healthy Carbs) or small garden salad

- ½ pound low-sodium turkey, rolled with 2 slices light or low-fat cheese, mustard, and optional peppers

- Innovation lunch meal (order online at innovationweightloss.com)

Dinner (Choose One)

- 10 ounces skinless grilled or rotisserie chicken or roast turkey

- 3 ounces shrimp or scallops, with 2 cups zucchini linguini mixed with 2 tablespoons Parmesan cheese and ¼ cup marinara sauce

- 10 ounces any baked or broiled fish or shellfish

- Innovation dinner meal (order online at innovationweightloss.com)

You can have an additional 3 cups of vegetables (see list under Rule 4, Healthy Carbs) with lunch or dinner each day, and one small sweet potato two times a week.

Snacks

The program allows three snacks per day, one from each category. If you don't want a snack from category 3, you can have a second snack from category 1 or 2, but never more than one snack from category 3. Snacks can be eaten in any order. You don't have to eat all the snacks. Less is more when trying to lose weight.

Category 1 (Choose One)

- 1 cup cut-up fruit or 1 piece of fruit (see list under Rule 4, Healthy Carbs)
- 1 small avocado with drizzle of lemon or lime juice

Category 2 (Choose One)

- 3 cups regular or sea salt, low-fat popcorn
- 1 cup vegetables with ¼ cup hummus
- 1 light cheese stick and 10 grapes
- Apple, with 1 tablespoon peanut butter or almond butter

Category 3 (Choose One)

- Innovation snack
- 1 cup fat-free chocolate pudding with 2 tablespoons whip cream or Cool Whip
- ¼ cup any plain, non-coated nuts (salted optional)
- 4 ounces wine or 1 ounce alcohol or 2 light beers

Drinks

- Unlimited water
- Coffee and tea (no sugar, but you can use artificial sweetener and a splash of skim milk)
- Diet drinks permitted

ON-PROGRAM FATS, HERBS, AND SPICES

Monounsaturated Fats	Herbs and Spices
Almond oil	Basil
Avocado	Cumin
Avocado oil	Garlic
Butter, mixed-nut butters	Lemon
Canola oil	Lime
Nuts and seeds	Mustard seeds
Olive oil	Onion
Peanut butter	Oregano
Almond butter	Paprika
Peanut oil	Parsley
Walnut oil	Pepper
	Sea salt
	Turmeric

RULE 7

FOLLOW THE INNOVATION PROGRAM FOR SUCCESS

I mentioned in the Introduction that one key to success with the *Innovation Weight Loss Program* is to start by reading the entire book. If you have not read the book from the beginning, you may gain some benefit, but will not cash in on the full benefit of the program. To implement the program successfully, it's important to learn and understand the *Cheat Day Rules!* Once you have read the entire book, then you can begin.

Step 1: Choose the menu (see Rule 6) that best suits you and your goals. This will be your base menu, and you will follow it six consecutive days each week.

Step 2: Choose which day of the week you want to begin the program. While Monday is often the choice for most people, you can start any day of the week. Remember, you have to have six or more on-program days before you take a Cheat Day. So if you start on Monday, your Cheat Day will be Sunday. You can change your Cheat Day every week, but it's important to always have at least six, full on-program days in-between. Factor this in when deciding what day you want to begin.

Step 3: Read through your menu and make sure you are prepared. Do your grocery shopping with your menu in hand so you have all the necessary foods and snacks you need. You don't ever want to be without the *Innovation Weight Loss Program* foods, or else you will grab and eat whatever is around.

Step 4: Once you choose your start day, weigh yourself that morning before you begin the program. If you want to use our Cheat Day Profile Page, sign onto cheatdayrules.com and log your weight every week, keeping track of your losses. You can also upload before-and-after photos or any photos that would help motivate you every day. On the Profile Page, you can also access our videos that will help you learn all about Cheat Day Rules as well as give you tips and helpful advice. Or you can listen to our podcasts, which include other clients sharing how they reached their goals on the Cheat Day

Rules program and what helped them the most.

If you choose not to use the Cheat Day Rules Profile Page, you can keep track of your weight in a notebook or pad. Start by writing the date and your starting weight. Remember, don't step on the scale until the morning of your Cheat Day.

Step 5: Every night, write down everything you ate and drank that day on your Profile Page or in your notebook. That way, at the end of the week or the end of the month, you can always look back to see what choices you made.

Step 6: Every day, make sure you are prepared with your meals and snacks. Remember that when midweek comes around and eating on program begins to feel a little challenging, your Cheat Day is only a couple of days away.

Step 7: Before you know it, your Cheat Day has arrived! Before you do anything, weigh yourself. Your new weigh-in day is the morning of every Cheat Day.

On your Cheat Day, you can choose to cheat all day or at a meal or just for dessert—the option is always yours. You can do the same thing every week or switch it up from week to week. The most important thing about the Cheat Day is to eat what you want, but always make sure you cheat *enough* so when your week starts again you feel satisfied. You can never do a Cheat Day wrong. Whatever you want to eat, whether you are eating all day or one meal, is up to you.

When to weigh yourself:

- First Weigh In—The day you begin
- Second Weigh In—The morning of your first Cheat Day (6 days from the first Weigh In)
- Continue Weighing—The morning of every weekly Cheat Day (at least 6 days apart)

Never weigh yourself *after* a Cheat Day since it takes your body time to process that day's food consumption.

RULE 8

REMEMBER HOW IMPORTANT SPECIAL OCCASIONS AND MAINTENANCE ARE TO CONTINUE ON YOUR HEALTHY PATH

O nce you reach your weight-loss goals, it can be difficult to maintain your new weight. For some people, maintenance can be harder than losing the weight. Below are some tips to help you maintain your new weight loss.

HOLIDAYS AND VACATIONS

So maybe you are in the middle of your weight-loss program (or have reached your goal), and a holiday is approaching. This might make you anxious. Even though you want to stay on program, being tempted could be too much. If you don't feel strong enough to get through the holiday on program, then use your Cheat Day. It's okay if you cheat midweek or not on your usual day. You just need to plan ahead and make sure to skip either the Cheat Day before or after the holiday to make up for the one holiday Cheat Day.

However, maybe you are one of the many people who realize they don't really like to use their Cheat Days for holidays. Well, you are not alone. Most clients don't like it because they find they are eating holiday foods, but not necessarily the foods they missed or feel satisfied with. If you choose not to use your Cheat Day, then you can stay on program and make sure that there is on-program food where you are celebrating. If it's back-to-back holidays (like Christmas Eve and Christmas Day), you always have the option of splitting the Cheat Day and eating on program all day (both days), but having only one meal and one dessert as Cheat meals for each day. But you must be prepared when you split the Cheat Day. You can only do it if it's back-to-back days, and you must be aware that you will not lose weight that week—you will only maintain. After you split Cheat Days, you need to go right back on program and have your next Cheat Day the following week or weekend.

Vacations can be a little challenging, usually because they are at least two or three days. You can do one of two things: Stay on program, making sure that wherever you are traveling, there will be foods that you can choose from to stay on program. Or you can do what many clients do—travel with your own snacks and bars so you have something to eat no matter where you are.

You may feel that, since it's your vacation, you just want to enjoy and not have to think about everything. But you still want to maintain weight. In that case, follow this plan: Every day, choose only one indulgence (whether it's a meal or dessert), then the rest of the day try to make choices that are as close to the program as you can. This will help you maintain—instead of gain—while on vacation.

DAILY MAINTENANCE

Congratulations! You've reached your weight-loss goal. So how do you maintain your achievement? Once you reach your goal, you should continue to stay on program for at least a month—six days on program, followed by one Cheat Day. If you find that you are still losing weight and want to stop, then it's time to do maintenance. There are two ways to do maintenance:

1. Three times a week, enjoy an extra on-program snack or add either ½ white potato, 1 small sweet potato, or ½ cup cooked rice to lunch or dinner. You still will have your once-a-week Cheat Day.

2. Stay on program five days and have two Cheat Days. Most clients prefer this approach because it gives them the freedom to enjoy their weekends without having to choose one day. Also, when you have two days, you might even eat less than trying to fit everything into one Cheat Day. Some people will cheat for one meal on one day, then do one full Cheat Day on the other, working their way to two full Cheat Days.

It doesn't have to be the same every week. But you can't do #1 *and* #2—it has to be one or the other. If you switch back and forth, then you need a regular on-program week in-between.

If you find that you start to struggle, simply go right back on program with your six on-program days, followed by one Cheat Day. Do this for a month straight and then try maintenance again.

FINAL THOUGHTS

I started the *Innovation Weight Loss Program* because I knew how difficult the struggle to lose weight can be. If you have ever tried to lose weight, it's likely you've spent a lot of time beating yourself up over the *forbidden* foods you ate. As soon as you ate something you *shouldn't have*, you probably regretted it and asked yourself, "Why did I do that? I messed up. What's the point?" The insults and recriminations you threw at yourself derailed your best intentions, no matter how much will power you may have had. That's why the *Innovation Weight Loss Program* includes Cheat Days. You follow the program for six days, and on the seventh, you can have your cake, pizza, pasta, potatoes, or whatever it is you crave.

With the *Innovation Weight Loss Program*, I have been able to help thousands of people go from being overweight, unhappy, and scared to becoming healthy, thin, and happy. It's amazing how losing weight with the program gave them new outlooks on life and put a jump back in their step.

For your first couple of Cheat Days, you'll probably overdo it and not feel so great the next day. Eventually you'll discover that you don't want to eat just to eat.

The differences between mental and physical hunger, wanting and needing food, will become clear. As a result, you will be successful, rather than deprived, on your weight-loss journey. Here are key things to remember if you want to lose weight:

- Eat clean and follow the *Innovation Weight Loss Program* for six consecutive days
- Include one Cheat Day once a week
- Do not skip your weekly Cheat Day

By following these guidelines, you'll lose weight and keep it off. Forever.

Remember, Cheat Day Rules!

ABOUT THE AUTHOR

Josephine Fitzpatrick began her career working as a private nutrition and weight-loss consultant, offering her clients 24/7 support and helping them find a healthier, cleaner way of life that they could maintain long term. As popularity for her approach grew, she launched innovationweightloss.com, offering personalized programs and individual support for thousands of people from all walks of life, including high-profile clients and A-list celebrities. Offices for innovationweightloss.com are located in Woodbury, Long Island, and in New York City. Josephine lives in New York with her husband, children, and dog.

INNOVATION WEIGHT LOSS PROGRAM

If you would like specific menus created for your personal weight-loss goals, visit innovationweight lossandfitness.com or cheatdayrules.com, and my team and I will personally work with you to create a weight-loss menu for your current weight, age, height, gender, lifestyle, and eating habits. We can provide gluten-free, dairy-free, vegetarian, or low-sugar/low-carb dietary plans.

To view and order Innovation foods and snacks, visit our website at innovationweightloss.com or cheatdayrules.com. At our website you can you use all the tools below or just those that you need:

- Register and create a profile page
- Track your weight loss
- Sign up for an individualized menu and support
- Sign up for 24/7 support only (if using menus from this book)
- Request add-ins (additional choices to your current menu)
- Read our blogs
- Listen to our Love to Live Healthy podcasts
- Watch our videos
- Shop in our Food Store, where we offer overnight shipping nationally

We want to make this as easy as you want it to be. We can hold your hand from beginning to end or just be there when you have a question or two. Whatever you decide, know that you will be thrilled with your weight-loss results.

RECIPES

**COMPLETE 4 WEEKS
ON PROGRAM BEFORE
ADDING ANY OF THE
FOLLOWING RECIPES**

MEALS

Slow Cooker Eggplant Italiano

Ingredients

1 large eggplant, sliced into half-inch discs

1 teaspoon garlic powder

1 teaspoon Italian seasoning

2 cups marinara sauce

1 cup shredded mozzarella cheese

Salt

Pepper

Directions

Place eggplant slices on paper-towel lined baking sheet and sprinkle both sides of each piece with salt. Let sit for 30 minutes and pat dry.

Spread about one-third of sauce in bottom of slow cooker. Season eggplant with garlic powder, Italian seasoning, and a dash of salt and pepper.

Arrange an even layer of eggplant slices into the slow cooker. Top with more sauce and a sprinkle of mozzarella cheese. Repeat layering two more times.

Cook on high for 4 to 5 hours.

6-ounce servings

Cauliflower Rice

Ingredients

3 garlic cloves, minced

1 medium onion diced

2 teaspoon olive oil

½ cup peas

1 cup string beans

¼ cup shredded carrots

1 cup egg whites scrambled (liquid egg whites, or whites of about 8 large eggs)

3 cups grated raw cauliflower

2 to 4 tablespoons liquid aminos or coconut aminos (healthy soy sauce alternative)

Directions

Heat pan on medium-high heat, sauté garlic and onions in 2 teaspoons olive oil until onions become soft.

Stir in peas, string beans, and carrots, and cook until vegetables are soft.

Add in the scrambled egg whites, cauliflower, and aminos.

Cook for about 4 to 7 minutes.

2 servings

Everything Chicken

Ingredients

¼ cup everything seeds, available in bagel shops, or a brand name blend, such as Trader Joe's Everything but the Bagel Sesame Seasoning Blend

4 6-ounce chicken cutlets

½ cup egg whites (liquid egg whites, or whites of about 4 large eggs)

Directions

Preheat oven to 425°F.

Line a baking sheet with tin foil.

Place ½ cup egg whites in a bowl and whisk them.

Dip the chicken in the egg whites, roll them in the everything seeds, then place on the baking sheet.

Bake the chicken at 425°F until thoroughly cooked (25–30 minutes).

4 servings

Oven Baked Blackened Tilapia

Ingredients

2 6-ounce tilapia fillets

2 teaspoons olive oil

2¼ tablespoon paprika

¾ teaspoon salt

¾ tablespoon onion powder

¾ teaspoon black pepper

½ teaspoon cayenne pepper (use sparingly, as it is super spicy!)

¾ teaspoon thyme

¾ teaspoon oregano

½ teaspoon garlic powder

Nonstick cooking spray

Directions

Preheat oven to 425°F.

In a bowl, combine spices together.

Line a sheet pan with foil and spray with nonstick cooking spray.

Rinse and pat fillets dry.

Brush each fillet with 1 teaspoon olive oil.

Cover the fillets with the spices and rub them in (both sides).

Arrange fillets on the pan and spray lightly with nonstick cooking spray.

Place pan in preheated oven.

Cook until nicely brown and flaky (9–11 minutes).

2 servings

Lemony Chicken Soup

Ingredients

1 bone-in whole chicken breast

4 whole carrots

1 lemon, sliced

4 sprigs fresh dill

4 sprigs fresh parsley

4 cups fat-free low-sodium chicken broth

8 ounces snap peas

2 cups water

Directions

Place chicken, carrots, and lemon in a 5–6 quart slow cooker.

Add in the dill and parsley and nestle it among the chicken and vegetables.

Add broth and 2 cups of water.

Cover and cook until chicken is cooked through and easily shreds (7–8 hours on low or 4–5 hours on high).

Thirty minutes before serving, transfer the chicken to a bowl and the carrots to a cutting board.

Discard the lemon and herbs.

Strain the liquid (if desired) and return to the slow cooker.

Cut carrots into rounds and shred the chicken into large pieces, discarding the bone.

Just before serving, return the chicken and carrots to the slow cooker, add in snaps peas and heat for 3 minutes.

2-cup servings

Egg White Salad

Ingredients

1 dozen egg whites (large eggs), hardboiled and chopped

3 stalks celery, finely chopped

½ red onion, finely chopped

2 tablespoons fresh dill, finely chopped

2 tablespoons light or low-fat mayonnaise

1 tablespoon lemon juice (about ½ fresh lemon)

1 tablespoon Dijon mustard

1 teaspoon paprika

Salt and pepper

Directions

In a large bowl, combine egg whites, celery, red onion, and dill.

In a small bowl, mix together mayo, lemon juice, mustard, and paprika.

Season to taste with salt and pepper.

Fold mayo mixture into bowl with egg whites using a rubber spatula.

½ lb. servings

Peaches and Cream Breakfast Smoothie

Ingredients

½ cup crushed ice (add more ice for a thicker smoothie)

1 cup unsweetened almond milk or skim milk

½ cup sliced peaches

1 scoop Quest Vanilla Milkshake Protein Powder

Directions

Mix together all ingredients into a blender and blend until smooth.

For a thicker consistency, add more ice.

1 serving

Spicy Turkey Burger

Ingredients

1 lb. lean ground turkey

2 cloves garlic, finely chopped

2 tablespoons chopped cilantro

½ red pepper, finely chopped

1 jalapeno pepper, finely chopped

2 teaspoons ground cumin

1 teaspoon chili powder

1 teaspoon salt

Directions

Combine all ingredients in bowl and divide mixture into four 4-ounce patties.

Heat a grill pan to medium heat and cook burgers until done (about 3 minutes per side).

4 servings

SNACKS

Frozen Peanut Butter Cups

Ingredients

½ cup peanut butter

12-ounce container of Cool Whip

2 tablespoons chocolate syrup

Directions

In a bowl, mix ½ cup peanut butter with one container of Cool Whip.

Fill muffin tin with cupcake liners.

Spoon mixture into muffin tin, filling each cup half full.

Drizzle with chocolate syrup.

Place in freezer for 6–8 hours before serving.

1 Peanut Butter Cup per serving

Baked "Apple Pie" Cups

Ingredients

2 Honeycrisp apples

½ tablespoon McCormick Apple Pie Spice seasoning

½ tablespoon vanilla extract

2 tablespoons Cool Whip

Directions

Preheat oven to 400°F.

Line a baking sheet with tinfoil.

Wash apples.

Slice about 1/3 off the top of the apple.

Core the apple and discard core and seeds.

Scoop out the center of the apple, and finely chop the apple pieces.

In a bowl, mix together the chopped apple pieces, apple pie seasoning, and ½ tablespoon vanilla extract.

Fill the apple shells with apple mixture and place on baking sheet.

Bake until apple mixture is tender (10–12 minutes).

Top each apple with 1 tablespoon Cool Whip.

2 servings